STOP!

DO NOT TAKE THAT SHOT!

BECAUSE VACCINES ARE SAFE!
DO YOU KNOW WHAT SAFE MEANS?

By (K.O.B) Kayy0hBee

This book is dedicated to: The thousands upon thousands of people who've suffered directly and indirectly from adverse/side effects of vaccines, including death, and those who have lost a loved one in connection to the COVID-19 pandemic. This book is also dedicated to Those of Limited Views [the people] by way of Great Alternative Virtues (G.A.V), an unincorporated organization, concerning information established in this book.

A notice to all: No information in this book is provided as legal advice, health care advice, or medical advice. One must always seek a competent attorney for legal advice and a certified health care professional who is licensed to provide medical care and health care advice. Because of sudden changes and advances in the laws, and

Introduction

This book may be small in size, but is well worth making it available to provide key insights into what we've never heard or seen described in such great details, prior to the publication of   "STOP! DO NOT TAKE THAT SHOT! BECAUSE VACCINES ARE SAFE!"

This small promotional book (SPB) is an extracted chapter taken from another book called "HOW COVID-19, VACCINES, TEST KITS AND THE WHOLE PANDEMIC STAND ON POLITICAL SCIENCE," by (K.O.B) Kayy0hBee.

The reader, when finish, will close this book feeling much more aware and want more information like this, and may want to consider purchasing the book in full, where this information was taken from called **"HOW COVID-19, VACCINES, TEST KITS AND THE WHOLE PANDEMIC STAND ON POLITICAL SCIENCE,"** by (K.O.B) Kayy0hBee.

Congratulations on the purchase, and know you will enjoy the read.

PART I: Are Vaccines Safe?

Like most people, I used to take everything at face value. Especially, if it was aired on the news or radio stations, from sales pitches, to promotions of government propaganda and advertisements that continues to flood the mainstream media. I believed in it all. Until the day I started to understand the correct usage of its language.

What Does "SAFE" actually Mean?

"Safe" is one of the most overlooked and possibly, the most dangerous word to be used in the promotions of encouraging people to become vaccinated. When politicians, bureaucrats, Judges, attorneys, or any other government officials of any branch is speaking, it would be more beneficial to understand their correct intentional meanings, oppose to one's own assumptions and presumptions.

If we draw back our attention to "The Ingraham Angle" from FOX NEWS back in April, 2020, Dr. Dan Erickson and Dr. Artin Massihi shared some very interesting insights into what doctors were being encouraged to do, during the pandemic and how "the California's stay-at-home- order" [mostly, all states] was lacking science.

What did they say, about *science* and the word *safe?*

The E.R. doctors had stated the following:

"It's interesting when I'm writing about my [patients] death report, I'm being pressured to add COVID. Why is that?"

"Something else is going on here. This is not about science and it's not even about COVID. When [authorities] use the word 'safe' -- if you listen to the word 'safe', that's about controlling you."

To help remove any forms of assumptions and presumptions when you hear the promotional or marketing phrase *"Vaccines are safe"* one can look toward the following information that was placed on the web page of Children's Hospital of Philadelphia. It simply states in the first paragraph:

"The first definition of the word safe is 'harmless.' This definition would imply that any negative consequence of a vaccine would make the vaccine unsafe. Using this definition, no vaccine is 100 percent safe. Almost all vaccines can cause pain, redness or tenderness at the site of injection. And some vaccines cause more severe side effects.

For example, the original pertussis (whooping cough) vaccine could cause persistent, inconsolable crying, high fever or seizures associated with fever. Although none of these severe symptoms resulted in permanent damage, they could be quite frightening to parents."

Let's explore how the word *safe* can be used, and then, look at some real-life examples.

When the CDC website claims, *"COVID-19 vaccines are **safe and effective; and severe reactions after vaccination are rare;"** then one should not assume their physical body and/or health is guaranteed to be safe from harm.

To help open the mind to other possible usages of the term "safe" compare the statements below and ask yourself the following question:

Are all the following statements saying the exact same thing, in a different way?

1) COVID-19 vaccines are safe.

2) Vaccines are safe.

3) Vaccines are safe, but not the person receiving the vaccines is safe.

4) Vaccines are safe and protected more so than the person receiving it.

5) Vaccines are unlikely to be overturned or proved wrong, no matter how many people suffers from adverse effects or vaccine injuries.

6) A clinical trial - Vaccines are *Safety After Fifty Evaluation (SAFE)*.

7) Vaccines are free from danger.

8) Vaccines are in a safe condition, *in its containers*.

9) Vaccines are secure from risk.

10) Vaccines are safe investments; a safe bet. *-As an investor.*

In Black's Law Dictionary Tenth Edition, the word *safe* has two definitions as an adjective and a third one in all capital letters, abbreviated.

The following definitions to *"safe"* are:

1) *Not exposed to danger; not causing danger.*

2) Unlikely to be overturned or proved wrong.

3) SAFE – means Sexual-assault forensic examiner.

Unless, one is claiming *there is no danger to the vaccines,* we can rule out the first definition, because no vaccines are 100 percent safe according to all vaccine inserts and according to the CDC website concerning COVID-19 vaccines. The CDC website states,

"Cases of myocarditis and pericarditis have rarely been observed following receipt of COVID-19 vaccines used in the United States. Evidence from multiple monitoring systems in the United States and around the globe support a causal association between mRNA COVID-19 vaccines (i.e., Moderna or Pfizer-BioNTech) and myocarditis and pericarditis."

"Myocarditis is inflammation of the heart muscle, and pericarditis is inflammation of the lining outside the heart; myopericarditis is present when both myocarditis and pericarditis occur at the same time. In these conditions, inflammation occurs in response to an infection or some other trigger."

"Cases of myocarditis and pericarditis have occurred most frequently in adolescent and young adult males within 7 days after receiving the second dose of an mRNA COVID-19 vaccine; however, cases have also been observed after dose 1 and booster doses."

The CDC also states:

"Adverse Events (Serious Safety Problems) Are Rare"

"In rare cases, people have experienced serious health events after COVID-19 vaccination. Any health problem that happens after vaccination is considered an adverse event.

An adverse event can be caused by the vaccine or can be caused by a coincidental event not related to the vaccine, such as an unrelated fever, that happened following vaccination."

"Anaphylaxis is a severe type of allergic reaction with symptoms such as hives, difficulty breathing, low blood pressure, or significant swelling of the tongue or lips. **Anaphylaxis after COVID-19 vaccination is rare.**"

Now, why would anyone place themselves or their children at any potential risks that are far more damaging and more dangerous than the actual disease one is trying to avoid?

Look at definition number #2 on the previous page, then ask yourself,

When is that definition actually used?

There was a news report video In January 2021 concerning a father *(Tim Zook)*, 60, who had died four days after receiving his second dose of the Pfizer's COVID vaccine.

At that time, it would appear more people were too afraid of speaking out loud their opinions to say what seemed to be the most obvious – *"the vaccines are more likely the cause, of all of these sudden deaths."*

Instead, no matter how many deaths and injuries following a vaccination, the vaccines seemed to always be given some extra credit of protection, and the benefit of doubt.

Sometimes, when the truth would be told, it would be given in such a way, as to attempt to **normalize vaccine injuries and deaths,** by saying it's very rare.

The term **"rare"** does not mean one is protected from suffering a vaccine injury, or death.

And no one ever asked, *how many vaccine injuries and deaths are needed, where it's no longer considered to be rare?*

A prime example of this normalization, was another death reported by Fox News : **Utah mother dies four days after taking second COVID-19 vaccine dose.**

"A 39-year-old Utah mom died just four days after receiving her second dose of the Moderna COVID-19 vaccine, according to a Wednesday report that investigated vaccine side effects.

Kassidi Kurill, who lived in Ogden, took the second dose on Monday, Feb. 1. By Friday evening that week, she was dead, according to 2News, which was the first to report on Kurill's case.

"She was seemingly healthy as a horse," Kurill's father, Alfred Hawley, told Fox News. "She had no known underlying conditions."

On Tuesday, Kurill's condition worsened. Her father said she complained that she was drinking fluids but not urinating and had a headache and nausea. By Wednesday, she felt a little better. But on Thursday, her heart began racing and Hawley took her to the hospital.

Kurill began throwing up. The doctors took blood tests, and she became less coherent, Hawley said. Thursday evening, she was transported to Trauma Center in Murray for a liver transplant.

Doctors tried repeatedly to stabilize her for a liver transplant but her condition deteriorated, and by Friday morning, she couldn't talk.

"They were trying to get her to a point where she was stable enough for a liver transplant. And they just could not get her stable," Hawley said. "She got worse and worse throughout the day. And at nine o'clock, she passed."

Without missing a beat, after reporting the death of this healthy 39-year-old mom, it was quickly followed up with the "**normalization of death,**" when it was concluded with the famous promotions of "**go-get-your-vaccine**" shot: In quotes:

"While side effects from the vaccine are common, resulting deaths are incredibly rare. According to the Center for Disease Control and Prevention's (CDC) Vaccine Adverse Event Reporting System (VAERS), some 92 million COVID-19 vaccine doses were administered in the U.S. between December 14, 2020 and March 8, 2021. Of those 92 million, VAERS received 1,637 reports of death (0.0018%) among people who received a COVID-19 vaccine.

"To date, VAERS has not detected patterns in cause of death that would indicate a safety problem with COVID-19 vaccines," the CDC says on its website.

Hawley, a civil servant and member of the National Guard, told Fox News he recognizes that his daughter's tragic death was one in a million.

"It appears she was the odd one out that had the terrible reaction," he said.

Despite his daughter's loss, Hawley, who is 69 years old and diabetic, said he has taken the vaccine himself because of the threat COVID-19 poses to his demographic.

*To those skeptical about taking the vaccine, Hawley said **"the vaccine is going to help you."***

"But if you have a reaction to it, don't ignore it. Don't be stoic and just say, 'Oh, I'll be fine,'" Hawley said. "Pay attention. If it persists beyond a day, you might ought to go see a doctor. And make sure that you're not another one in a million."

It's as if they are saying to everyone,

"Don't worry if it causes death, or some other types of serious injuries, because the benefits still outweigh the risks!"

And this is true from the position of the investors.

"Vaccines are safe!"

But this usage of *safe* does **not** mean an individual man, woman or child is protected from harm after "any" vaccination.

It would be very naïve to think otherwise, after reading all of the Food and Drug Administration Package Inserts and **Bruesewitz v. Wyeth LLC, 562 U.S. 223 (2011),** from JUSTIA U.S. Supreme Court, which states, in part:

Hannah Bruesewitz's parents filed a vaccine-injury petition in the Court of Federal Claims, claiming that Hannah became disabled after receiving a diphtheria, tetanus, and pertussis (DTP) vaccine manufactured by Lederle Laboratories (now owned by respondent Wyeth).

After that court denied their claim, they elected to reject the unfavorable judgment and filed suit in Pennsylvania state court, alleging, inter alia, that the defective design of Lederle's DTP vaccine caused Hannah's disabilities, and that Lederle was subject to strict liability and liability for negligent design under Pennsylvania common law.

Wyeth removed the suit to the Federal District Court. It granted Wyeth summary judgment, holding that the relevant Pennsylvania law was preempted by 42 U. S. C. §300aa–22(b)(1), which provides that "[n]o vaccine manufacturer shall be liable in a civil action for damages arising from a vaccine-related injury or death associated with the administration of a vaccine after October 1, 1988, if the injury or death resulted from side-effects that were unavoidable even though the vaccine was properly prepared and was accompanied by proper directions and warnings." The Third Circuit affirmed.

If it be true that *"[n]o vaccine manufacturer shall be liable in a civil action for damages arising from a vaccine-related injury or death associated with the administration of a vaccine after October 1, 1988, if the injury or death resulted from side-effects that were unavoidable even though the vaccine was properly prepared and was accompanied by proper directions and warnings,"* then the one only logical explanation that can be made is:

"The vaccines are safe, but NOT the person who's receiving the vaccines are safe from any vaccine injury or death related to the vaccines."

One sincerely held belief of Great Alternative Virtues (G.A.V) is, using vaccines is like playing Russian Roulette.

This nonprofit/private group G.A.V was created and funded by its own supporters which are valued members guaranteeing it to remain private without using government support. Their tenets qualify them for religious exemptions when it comes to vaccinations.

One of the disciplines or tenets of G.A.V concerning flu-shots, and vaccines in general, that was stated to its members was:

"Receiving the flu-shots or vaccines of any kind is like gambling and playing Russian-roulette with the individuals health and life."

"This goes against self-preservation, in which self-preservation is one of the most important tenets of G.A.V."

The number one Drug Tenet of G.A.V is:

"There is no reason for an individual who's not sick, ill, and doesn't have a disease of some kind, to receive any drugs or vaccinations; unless, it's given by prescription directly from the individuals licensed doctor. For an example, a family doctor might prescribe some prescription drug or medicine for a disease that was diagnosed; or some type of drug medication for pain after surgery."

Another sincerely held belief of G.A.V:,

"Everyone deserves the freedom of choice without coercion. Especially, when it's related to an individual's personal health; which is always private."

G.A.V promotes knowledge over belief (K.O.B) as their spiritual practice & lifestyle, while using reputable sources:

"Most people believe flu vaccinations are **safe,** so allow me to show you how **safe** they are.

Vaccines are so safe that there's a **Vaccine Injury Table** chart created and made available by government agencies: https://www.hrsa.gov/sites/default/files/hrsa/vicp/vaccine -injury-table-01-03-2022.pdf."

I'll keep it sweet and simple with 9 main points, and do not be disturbed by certain words you may not be familiar with, as it will become self-explanatory by the time you've reached the end.

1) Campylobacter infection is the most commonly identified cause of Guillan-Barré syndrome, according to the CDC. https://www.cdc.gov/campylobacter/index.html

2) Campylobacter causes an estimated 1.5 million illnesses each year in the United States; according to the web link.

3) One possible cause is that flu vaccine contains Campylobacter, said Dr Chen, of the CDC's immunization safety branch. He said that the vaccine is made in chicken eggs and that 40-50% of chickens are infected with Campylobacter, which is difficult to eradicate: https://www.ncbi.nlm.nih.gov/pmc/articles/PMC1169311

4) According to the Centers for Disease Control and Prevention (CDC) website, vaccine is associated with contributing factors that causes (GBS).

5) Guillain-Barré syndrome (GBS) is a rare disorder in which a person's own immune system damages their nerve cells, causing muscle weakness and sometimes paralysis.

6) GBS can cause symptoms that usually last for a few weeks. Most people recover fully from GBS, but some people have long-term nerve damage. In very rare cases, people have died of GBS, usually from difficulty breathing. In the United States, an estimated 3,000 to 6,000 people develop GBS each year.

7) People also can develop GBS after having the flu or other infections (such as cytomegalovirus and Epstein Barr virus).

8) It's claimed, on very rare occasions, people may develop GBS in the days or weeks after getting a vaccination.
See https://www.cdc.gov/flu/prevent/guillainbarre.htm

9) Anyone can develop GBS; however, it is more common among older adults. The incidence of GBS increases with age, and people older than 50 years are at greatest risk for developing GBS.

Now can you see how people's minds have been manipulated into thinking it's okay, for 3,000 to 6,000 to develop GBS, in just the United States alone?

The tendency to always say it's RARE is the process of normalizing an unfortunate event concerning vaccine injuries. And vaccines are NOT the best form of protection, according to Dr. Fauci's statement on record, in video form,

https://ugetube.com/embed/Qp7tNaxCP1g7iaU

And this is how **safe** the flu vaccines are."

https://ugetube.com/embed/KMv81rUnZMTnplT

There is no vaccine to better serve you, than your own immune system. If you have a healthy immune system, then you're already protected from the disease, without unwarranted risks of *common side effects* or any other *adverse events* from the use of a vaccine.

Any Other Definition of SAFE?

"YES!" It is only fitting to bring forth another definition as we've been reviewing the term *safe* and SAFE.

Although, it may or may not be as significant for some, I did start off by introducing you to the fact that there are multiple interpretations or usages, so why not know them all?

According to McGraw-Hill Concise Dictionary of Modern Medicine, the term "SAFE" as an abbreviation is as follows:

"In Cardiology A clinical trial – Safety After Fifty Evaluation [SAFE]."

The Safety After Fifty Evaluation trial was designed to determine the short-term efficacy and tolerability of once-daily therapy with the cardio selective [beta]-blocker metoprolol, any one, or in combination with hydrochlorothiazide in the treatment of mild hypertension in patients 50 to 75 years of age. A total of 24,816 patients were enrolled in the trial, by 2821 practicing physicians from across the United States.

In this sense, "SAFE" means Safety After Fifty Evaluation [trial].

As there are many famous quotes to mention, I'll leave you with this one to ponder on, by Sir William Osler.

"The good physician treats the disease; [While] the great physician treats the patient who has the disease
-Sir William Osler

Which physician would you prefer?

And which one do you currently have?

To the Reader

If you've enjoyed this type of read, you may want to enjoy a longer read and consider purchasing the book in full, **"HOW COVID-19, VACCINES, TEST KITS AND THE WHOLE PANDEMIC STAND ON POLITICAL SCIENCE,"** by (K.O.B) Kayy0hBee.

The book is broken into two main parts, consisting of 5 informative chapters, with subchapters, detailing how political science was used as the key factor to manifest a desired outcome, the names of the individuals and groups that were behind it, how many years in advance the pandemic was planned, the real history of corona viruses, and *possible solutions* based on how some people have used different remedies to protect themselves against forced vaccinations, while maintaining their jobs, or going to school. These are topics not clearly spoken about in mainstream media, but you can read it in a book called:

"HOW COVID-19, VACCINES, TEST KITS AND THE WHOLE PANDEMIC STAND ON POLITICAL SCIENCE," by (K.O.B) Kayy0hBee.

Bibliography

Creitz C. (April 28, 2020) California urgent care doctor questions stay-at-home orders: 'You can get to herd immunity without a vaccine' https://www.foxnews.com/media/california-doctor-questions-stay-at-home-orders.

Offit P. MD (May 19, 2020) Children's Hospital of Philadelphia https://www.chop.edu/centers-programs/vaccine-education-center/vaccine-safety/are-vaccines-safe.

National Center for Immunization and Respiratory Diseases (NCIRD), Division of Viral Diseases (Updated Mar. 7, 2023) https://www.cdc.gov/coronavirus/2019-ncov/vaccines/safety/safety-of-vaccines.html.

National Center for Immunization and Respiratory Diseases (March 23, 2023) Clinical Considerations: Myocarditis and Pericarditis after Receipt of COVID-19 Vaccines Among Adolescents and Young Adults https://www.cdc.gov/vaccines/covid-19/clinical-considerations/myocarditis.html.

Garner B. (2009) Black's Law Dictionary Tenth Edition. BMJ 2003; 326 doi: https://doi.org/10.1136/bmj.326.7390.620/b (Published 22 March 2003) https://www.ncbi.nlm.nih.gov/pmc/articles/PMC1169311/.

National Center for Immunization and Respiratory Diseases (March 7, 2023) Adverse Events (Serious Safety Problems) Are Rare https://www.cdc.gov/coronavirus/2019-ncov/vaccines/safety/safety-of-vaccines.html.

Centers for Disease Control and Prevention, National Center for Immunization and Respiratory Diseases (NCIRD) (October 16, 2015) "Guillain-Barré syndrome and Flu Vaccine" https://www.cdc.gov/flu/prevent/guillainbarre.htm.

The CDC (April 14. 2021) Campylobacter (Campylobacteriosis) https://www.cdc.gov/campylobacter/index.html.

SANTA ANA (CBSLA)/KCAL NEWS LOS ANGELES (January 28,2021) 60-Year-Old Father Dies After Receiving Second Dose Of Pfizer Vaccine https://www.cbsnews.com/losangeles/news/pfizer-vaccine-orange-county-moderna/.

Betz B. FoxNews Channel (March 10, 2021) "Utah mother dies four days after taking second COVID-19 vaccine dose" https://www.foxnews.com/us/utah-mom-dies-four-days-after-taking-covid-vaccine.

Hatch H. (March 10th 2021)"ME says vaccine not cause of Utah Woman's Death After 2nd dose" https://kutv.com/news/local/utah-woman-39-dies-4-days-after-2nd-does-of-covid-19-vaccine-autopsy-ordered.

JUSTIA U.S. Supreme Court (2011) Bruesewitz v. Wyeth LLC, 562 U.S. 223 https://supreme.justia.com/cases/federal/us/562/223/.

Rich M.; LaPalio L.; Schork A.; SAFE Coordinators (1988/07) The Safety After Fifty Evaluation trial: Evaluation of the safety and efficacy of antihypertensive therapy with metoprolol in patients 50 to 75 years of age: Study design. https://deepblue.lib.umich.edu/handle/2027.42/27529.

Acknowledgements

A special acknowledgement to all of the professionals, content creators, researchers, and all other people who realized the true facts; and shared that information even when it wasn't so popular to do so.

Some of these people are still doing great work like, Dr. Artin Massihi, Dr. Dan Erickson, Dr. Scott Jensen, James Corbett, Redacted - with Natali and Clayton Morris, SquirrelTribe, EnQurrios and many others, whose names are not mentioned here.

Dr. Shiva and High Frequency Radio (Yusef El) are two of the most inspiring people who shouldn't be overlooked, for all of the years of consistency in providing quality information. A big huge thanks to Unincorporated Thoughts for the videos researched and supporting of our work, and Great Alternative Virtues (G.A.V) for creating our logos, picture editing and modifications, while sharing researched materials with knowledge over belief and appointing us as their original sole spokesperson for publications and communications [of their work]

Other Special Thanks to: Maria Origel and Chuck Quiring – two great spirited people who've always encouraged and supported the ideas of the production of books; John Hudson, who's a very strong supporter for the opposing side, helped indirectly to conjure this book; Fannie Green (who gave so much while she was here and is forever loved and missed), and other inspirations: G. Pearl, Brian Jefferson, David Haynes, Jerry Wilson, Don Khamsingsavath, and last but not least Sheila Wright.

About the Author

Over 26 years of hospital experience in two different institutions, with special interests as an examiner of investigational studies and research, medical terminology, legal research and terminology, and law.

www.ingramcontent.com/pod-product-compliance
Lightning Source LLC
Chambersburg PA
CBHW060019300526
45794CB00003B/1219